W9-BUJ-249

Workbook to Accompany

MOSBY'S

Canadian

Textbook

for the

Support

Worker

Second Canadian Edition

evolve

⠆⠆ To access your Student Resources, visit the web address below:

http://evolve.elsevier.com/Canada/Sorrentino/SupportWorker

Evolve® Student Resources for *Mosby's Canadian Textbook for the Support Worker,* **Second Edition,** offer the following features:

Student Resources

- **Content Updates**
  Provide updates to textbook content.

- **Checklists**
  Allow for self-examination.

- **Audio Glossary**
  Provides definitions of key terms in addition to audio pronunciations for selected key terms.

- **Body Spectrum**
  Provides interactive review of Anatomy and Physiology content.

- **Skills Evaluation**
  Allows for self-examination on performing procedures.

- **Video Clips**
  Demonstrate important steps in procedures included in the textbook.

http://evolve.elsevier.com/Canada/Sorrentino/SupportWorker

Workbook to Accompany

MOSBY'S

Canadian Textbook for the Support Worker

RELDA TIMMENLY KELLY
RN, BSN, MSN
Instructor
Kankalee Community College

SHEILA A. SORRENTINO
RN, PhD
Curriculum and Health Care Consultant
Normal, Illinois

CANADIAN AUTHORS
Rosemary Newmaster, *RN*
Instructor and Coordinator, Personal Support Worker Program, Fleming College
Mary J. Wilk, *RN, GNC(C), BA, BScN, MN(c)*
Professor & Coordinator, Personal Support Program, Fanshawe College

Second Canadian Edition

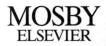

MOSBY
ELSEVIER

Copyright © 2009 Elsevier Canada, a division of Reed Elsevier Canada, Ltd.

All rights reserved. No part of this publication may be reproduced or transmitted in any form or by any means, electronic or mechanical, including photocopy, recording, or any information storage and retrieval system without permission in writing from the publisher. Reproducing passages from this book without such written permission is an infringement of copyright law.

Requests for permissions to make copies of any part of the work should be mailed to: College Licensing Officer, access ©, 1Yonge Street, Suite 1900, Toronto, ON M5E 1E5.

Every reasonable effort has been made to acquire permission for copyright material used in this text and to acknowledge all such indebtedness accurately. Any errors and omissions called to the publisher's attention will be corrected in future printings.

Library and Archives Canada Cataloguing in Publication

Sorrentino, Sheila A.
    Workbook to accompany Mosby's Canadian textbook for the support worker / Sheila Sorrentino, Mary J. Wilk, Rosemary Newmaster. — 2nd Canadian ed.

ISBN 978-0-7796-9944-5

    1. Nurses' aides—Problems, exercises, etc. 2. Care of the sick—Problems, exercises, etc. I. Newmaster, Rosemary. II. Wilk, Mary J. III. Title.

RT84.S67 2008 Suppl.   610.7306'98   C2007-902089-5

VP, Publishing: Ann Millar
Managing Developmental Editor: Martina van de Velde
Developmental Editor: Toni Chahley
Managing Production Editor: Rohini Herbert
Copy Editor: Holly Dickinson
Cover Design: Olena Sullivan/New Mediatrix
Typesetting and Assembly: Jansom
Printing and Binding: Transcontinental

Elsevier Canada
905 King Street West, 4th Floor
Toronto, ON, Canada M6K 3G9
Phone: 1-866-896-3331
Fax: 1-866-359-9534

Printed in Canada

2 3 4 5   13 12 11 10 09

Working together to grow libraries in developing countries

www.elsevier.com | www.bookaid.org | www.sabre.org

ELSEVIER   BOOK AID International   Sabre Foundation

"I would like to dedicate this workbook to all of my colleagues at Fanshawe College, as a testament to their support, assistance, and friendship. Thank you!"

Mary Wilk

"I would like to dedicate this workbook to all of my colleagues at Fleming College, as a testament to their support, assistance, and friendship. Thank you!"

Rosemary Newmaster

Contents

Introduction

This Workbook is intended to be used with *Mosby's Canadian Textbook for the Support Worker*, 2nd Canadian Edition. Additional resources are not required to complete the exercises in this Workbook.

This Workbook is designed as a study guide to help you apply what you have learned in each chapter of the textbook. As a supplementary to this Workbook, procedure checklists are featured on the Evolve Web site for *Mosby's Canadian Textbook for the Support Worker,* 2nd Canadian Edition. These checklists are designed to help you become more skilled at performing procedures to enhance the quality of care. Consult with your instructor for correct answers to material presented in this Workbook and on the Evolve Web site's procedure checklists. The Evolve Web site for *Mosby's Canadian Textbook for the Support Worker*, 2nd Canadian Edition, can be accessed at http://evolve.elsevier.com/Canada/Sorrentino/SupportWorker/.

As a support worker, you are an important member of the health care team. Completing the exercises in this Workbook will increase your knowledge and skills. Our goal is to prepare you to provide the best possible care to your clients and to encourage you to take pride in a job well done.

TRUE OR FALSE

Circle T for true or F for false. Rewrite all false statements to make them true. The statements apply to rules for recording.

1. **T**   **F**   Write notes in pencil.

   _____

   _____

2. **T**   **F**   Include the date whenever a recording is made.

   _____

   _____

3. **T**   **F**   Make sure the writing is legible and neat.

   _____

   _____

4. **T**   **F**   Use any abbreviations needed to shorten an entry.

   _____

   _____

5. **T**   **F**   Use correct spelling, grammar, and punctuation.

   _____

   _____

6. **T**   **F**   Use an eraser or correction fluid if you make an error.

   _____

   _____

7. **T**   **F**   Sign all entries with your name and title as required by the agency.

   _____

   _____

8. **T**   **F**   Skip lines between entries.

   _____

   _____

9. **T**   **F**   Make sure each form is stamped with the person's name.

   _____

   _____

10. **T**   **F**   Record what you or others did or observed.

   _____

   _____

11. **T**   **F**   Chart all care and treatments early in the shift before beginning work.

   _____

   _____

12. **T**   **F**   Record your observations, interpretations, and judgements.

   _____

   _____

13. **T**   **F**   Record in a logical and sequential manner.

   _____

   _____

14. **T   F**   Avoid terms with more than one meaning.

_____

_____

15. **T   F**   Paraphrase the client's words to make the meaning more understandable.

_____

_____

16. **T   F**   Chart any changes from normal or changes in the client's condition.

_____

_____

17. **T   F**   Omit unimportant information.

_____

_____

18. **T   F**   Record safety measures used in caring for the client.

_____

_____

FILL-IN-THE-BLANKS

19. What are the four senses you use to obtain information about a client?

a. _____

b. _____

c. _____

d. _____

20. When a client reports things you cannot observe by using your senses, they are called symptoms or _____

_____ data.

21. When you can obtain information about a client with your senses, it is called signs or

_____

_____ data.

22. The following words or phrases are either subjective or objective data. In the blank next to each one, place an "S" for subjective or an "O" for objective.

a. _____   Sleepy

b. _____   Chest pain

c. _____   Skin cool

d. _____   Bruises

e. _____   Difficulty breathing

f. _____   Gas pain

g. _____   Pain when urinating

h. _____   Productive cough

i. _____   Breath has a fruity odour

j. _____   Rapid pulse and shallow breathing

23. The following statements are either subjective or objective. Place an "S" for a subjective statement or an "O" for an objective statement.

a. _____   Mr. Jones states that he is cold.

b. _____   Mary has red hair.

c. _____   Mrs. Smith says she has pain in her right shoulder.

d. _____   Temperature 37.6°C (99.6°F), pulse 72, respirations 16

e. _____ Mr. Green ate all of his breakfast.

f. _____ Mrs. Foster says she is anxious about having surgery.

24. What are the four senses you use to obtain information about a client?

  a. _____

  b. _____

  c. _____

  d. _____

25. Next to each of the following, write the time using the 24-hour clock.

  a. _____ 11:00 A.M.   g. _____ 3:00 A.M.

  b. _____ 8:00 A.M.   h. _____ 4:50 A.M.

  c. _____ 4:00 P.M.   i. _____ 5:30 P.M.

  d. _____ 7:30 A.M.   j. _____ 10:45 P.M.

  e. _____ 6:45 P.M.   k. _____ 11:55 P.M.

  f. _____ 12 noon   l. _____ 9:15 P.M.

26. When you write entries in the chart, you

  sign your name and _____ .

27. What basic observations will give you information about a client?

  a. _____

  b. _____

  c. _____

  d. _____

  e. _____

  f. _____

  g. _____

h. _____

i. _____

28. What basic observations can you make to determine a client's ability to respond?

  a. _____

  b. _____

  c. _____

  d. _____

  e. _____

  f. _____

  g. _____

  h. _____

29. What observations will help to determine whether a client has normal movement?

  a. _____

  b. _____

  c. _____

  d. _____

30. What words help a client to describe his or her pain?

  a. _____

  b. _____

  c. _____

  d. _____

  e. _____

  f. _____

  g. _____

  h. _____

31. What observations should be made about a client's respirations?

    a. _____

    b. _____

    c. _____

    d. _____

    e. _____

32. When observing the skin, what questions should be asked?

    a. _____

    b. _____

    c. _____

    d. _____

    e. _____

    f. _____

    g. _____

    h. _____

33. What observations are important to determine how the bowels and bladder are functioning?

    a. _____

    b. _____

    c. _____

    d. _____

    e. _____

    f. _____

    g. _____

    h. _____

    i. _____

    j. _____

34. What activities of daily living should be observed?

    a. _____

    b. _____

    c. _____

    d. _____

    e. _____

35. When reporting to the nurse, you should:

    a. be _____, _____,

       and _____ .

    b. tell the nurse the client's _____,

       _____, and _____ .

    c. report only _____ .

    d. give reports as often as _____

       _____ .

    e. immediately report _____

       _____ .

    f. use progress notes to record _____

       _____ .

36. Use the chart as a guide and convert the following times. Convert **a** through **d** from conventional time to the 24-hour clock. Convert **e** through **h** from the 24-hour clock to conventional time.

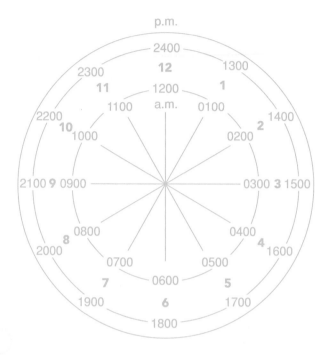

a. 2:00 A.M. = _____

b. 10:30 A.M. = _____

c. 5:00 A.M. = _____

d. 9:30 A.M. = _____

e. 0600 = _____ A.M.   P.M.
         (circle one)

f. 1145 = _____ A.M.   P.M.
         (circle one)

g. 1800 = _____ A.M.   P.M.
         (circle one)

h. 2200 = _____ A.M.   P.M.
         (circle one)

MULTIPLE CHOICE

Circle the correct answer.

37. Which of these is not a rule of communication?
    a. Use words that have only one meaning.
    b. Give a very detailed and lengthy explanation.
    c. Be specific and concise when giving information.
    d. Organize information in a logical manner.

38. What information is not included on the graphic sheet?
    a. Temperature, pulse, respirations
    b. Bowel sounds
    c. Height and weight
    d. Bowel movements

39. The Kardex is a:
    a. part of the medical record (chart).
    b. sheet used to record measurements or observations.
    c. written description of nursing care given.
    d. summary of treatments, diagnosis, and routine care measures.

40. Which of these is a question about an activity of daily living?
    a. Can the client perform personal care without help?
    b. How much food on the tray is eaten?
    c. What is the frequency of bowel movements?
    d. Can the client move arms and legs?

41. A purpose of a team meeting is to:
    a. identify the medical diagnosis.
    b. develop or revise a client's nursing care plan for effective care.
    c. share the end-of-shift report.
    d. chart day-to-day care of the client.

MATCHING

Match the following statements with one of the key terms related to communication.

42. _____ Identification of a disease or condition by a doctor

43. _____ Determining if the goals in the care plan have been met

44. _____ Statement describing a health problem that can be treated by nursing measures

45. _____ Written guide that gives direction about the care and services a client should receive

46. _____ Method used by nurses to plan and deliver nursing care

47. _____ Action taken by a nursing team member to help the client reach a goal

a. Nursing care plan

b. Nursing diagnosis

c. Nursing intervention

d. Care planning process

e. Medical diagnosis

f. Evaluation

Managing Stress, Time, and Problems

TRUE OR FALSE

Circle T for true or F for false. Rewrite all false statements to make them true.

1. **T**   **F**   Stressors over a short period of time can cause a chronic illness.

   _____

   _____

2. **T**   **F**   You should set weekly goals for yourself.

   _____

   _____

3. **T**   **F**   Getting a promotion can cause stress.

   _____

   _____

4. **T**   **F**   A child usually shows different signs of stress than an adult.

   _____

   _____

5. **T**   **F**   Time management is essential to reducing stress.

   _____

   _____

6. **T**   **F**   There is no point in planning your work a day ahead since things change when you get to work.

   _____

   _____

7. **T**   **F**   You don't need to report a conflict with a client if it is resolved.

   _____

   _____

8. **T**   **F**   In a home care setting, you must plan your time so you can be on time for the next client.

   _____

   _____

9. **T**   **F**   Older adults are less able to cope with stress.

   _____

   _____

10. **T**   **F**   All stress is bad for your well-being.

   _____

   _____

FILL-IN-THE-BLANKS

11. How can you manage stress in your life?

    a. _____

    b. _____

    c. _____

    d. _____

12. Problem solving is a process. Describe this process.

    _____

    _____

    _____

    _____

    _____

13. How can you save time and stay organized?

    a. _____

    b. _____

    c. _____

    d. _____

14. What can you do to manage conflict at work?

    a. _____

    b. _____

    c. _____

    d. _____

    e. _____

    f. _____

    g. _____

15. What are some common stressors you may face?

    a. _____

    b. _____

    c. _____

    d. _____

    e. _____

16. Physical signs of stress can be:

    a. _____ .

    b. _____ .

    c. _____ .

    d. _____ .

    e. _____ .

17. Emotional and behavioural signs of stress can include:

    a. _____ .

    b. _____ .

    c. _____ .

    d. _____ .

    e. _____ .

    f. _____ .

Growth and Development

TRUE OR FALSE

Circle T for true or F for false. Rewrite all false statements to make them true.

1. **T** **F** Three-month-old infants can raise their heads and shoulders when lying on their stomachs.

   _____

   _____

2. **T** **F** Toilet training is usually completed by the age of 1$^1/_2$ years.

   _____

   _____

3. **T** **F** Three-year-olds are able to play with other children.

   _____

   _____

4. **T** **F** Young adulthood is the time when partners spend more time alone together.

   _____

   _____

5. **T** **F** Adolescents begin to think about careers and what to do after high school graduation.

   _____

   _____

FILL-IN-THE-BLANKS

According to your textbook, at what age is a child expected to develop each of the following skills?

6. _____ Speaks in short sentences

7. _____ Usually protective of younger brothers and sisters

8. _____ Learns to write rather than print

9. _____ Smiles and follows objects with the eyes

10. _____ Can eat table food

11. _____ Capable of bladder control during the day

12. _____ Can hold a rattle

13. _____ Knows male and female bodies are different

14. _____ Reacts to the word "no"

15. _____ Begins to bite and chew finger foods

16. _____ Plays with the toes

17. What are the six basic principles of growth and development?

a. _____

_____

b. _____

_____

c. _____

_____

d. _____

_____

e. _____

_____

f. _____

_____

18. Physical changes that can be measured and occur in a steady and organized manner are

called _____

_____ .

19. A change in psychological and social

functioning is called _____

_____ .

20. A _____
is a baby in the first 4 weeks after birth.

21. The 4-year-old child has a strong preference

for the parent of the _____ sex.

22. At what age are peer-group activities and opinions important to the child?

_____

23. Adolescence begins when reproductive organs begin to function. What is this event called?

_____

24. During _____ ,
hobbies and pastimes can be pursued as more free time is available.

25. What stage of growth and development includes the following developmental tasks?

_____

• Adjusting to physical changes
• Having grown children
• Developing leisure-time activities
• Relating to aging parents

26. What stage of growth and development includes the following developmental tasks?

_____

• Increasing the ability to communicate and understand others
• Performing self-care activities
• Learning the differences between the sexes and developing sexual modesty
• Learning right from wrong and good from bad
• Learning to play with others
• Developing family relationships

Identify the age when each behaviour or physical change usually occurs.

27. _____ Do not like being teased or criticized and are sensitive about how others treat them

28. _____ Temper tantrums and saying "no" are common

29. _____ In girls, pelvis becomes broader, fat appears on hips and chest, and budding of breasts occurs

30. _____ Movements are uncoordinated and lack purpose

31. _____ Select partner and learn to live together, develop intimate relationships

32. _____ May be able to stand when holding onto something

33. _____ Menarche occurs, breasts increase in size, hair appears in pubic and axillary areas

34. _____ Bowel training usually is complete

35. _____ Awkward movements occur because of rapid growth in height and weight

36. _____ Recognizes that male and female bodies are different

37. _____ More permanent teeth appear; movements are faster and more graceful

38. _____ Weight control becomes a problem as metabolism and physical activity slow down

39. _____ May cheat to win, but they like rules and try to follow them

40. _____ Responsible for aging parents and deals with death of parents

41. _____ Makes decision to have children and plans number of children

42. _____ Baby teeth are lost, and replacement with permanent teeth begins

MULTIPLE CHOICE

Circle the correct answer.

43. The stage of infancy is the first:
    a. 4 weeks of life.
    b. 3 months of life.
    c. 6 months of life.
    d. first year of life.

44. Which reflexes are needed for feeding in the infant?
    a. the Moro and startle reflexes
    b. the rooting and sucking reflexes
    c. the grasping and Moro reflexes
    d. the rooting and grasping reflexes

45. Solid foods are usually given to an infant during the:
    a. fifth to seventh month.
    b. eighth month.
    c. ninth or tenth month.
    d. eleventh or twelfth month.

46. The toddler can:
    a. use a spoon and cup.
    b. ride a bike.
    c. help set the table.
    d. name parts of the body.

47. Playing with other children begins during:
    a. infancy.
    b. the toddler years.
    c. the preschool years.
    d. middle childhood.

48. Reproductive organs begin to function and secondary sex characteristics appear during:
    a. late childhood.
    b. preadolescence.
    c. puberty.
    d. early adulthood.

49. Middle adulthood is from about:
    a. 25 to 35 years.
    b. 30 to 40 years.
    c. 40 to 50 years.
    d. 40 to 65 years.

50. Middle adulthood is usually a time when:
    a. families are started.
    b. physical energy and free time are gained.
    c. children are grown and leave home.
    d. people need to prepare for death.

MATCHING

Match the following statements with the correct reflex of an infant. You can use a reflex more than once to answer.

51. _____ Produced by touching the cheeks

52. _____ When cheek is touched, baby turns head in the direction of touch

53. _____ A loud noise causes infant to throw arms apart and extend legs

54. _____ When palm of hand is touched, baby closes fingers around object

55. _____ Guides baby's mouth to nipple

56. _____ Disappears by the fourth month

a. Moro (startle) reflex

b. Rooting reflex

c. Sucking reflex

d. Grasping reflex

Match the developmental task with the correct age group. You can use an age group more than once to answer.

57. _____ Accepting the changes in body and appearance

58. _____ Developing leisure-time activities

59. _____ Gaining control of bowel and bladder functions

60. _____ Becoming independent from parents and adults

61. _____ Learning to eat solid foods

62. _____ Developing new friends and relationships

63. _____ Learning how to study

64. _____ Learning to get along with peers

65. _____ Increasing ability to communicate and understand others

66. _____ Tolerating separation from primary caregiver

67. _____ Learning to live with a partner

68. _____ Developing moral and ethical behaviour

69. _____ Learning basic reading, writing, and arithmetic skills

70. _____ Developing stable sleep and feeding patterns

71. _____ Performing self-care activities

72. _____ Using words to communicate with others

73. _____ Relating to aging parents

74. _____ Accepting male or female role appropriate for one's age

75. _____ Beginning to have emotional relationships with primary caregivers, brothers, and sisters

a. Infancy (birth to 1 year)

b. Toddler (1 to 3 years)

c. Preschooler (3 to 6 years)

d. Middle childhood (6 to 8 years)

e. Late childhood (9 to 12 years)

f. Adolescence (12 to 18 years)

g. Young adulthood (18 to 40 years)

h. Middle adulthood (40 to 65 years)

i. Late adulthood (65 years and older)

Caring for the Young

TRUE OR FALSE

Circle T for true or F for false. Rewrite all false statements to make them true.

1. **T** **F** Do not tie pacifiers or other items around a baby's neck.

   _____

   _____

2. **T** **F** Position infants on their stomach in the crib.

   _____

   _____

3. **T** **F** It is not your duty to provide a stable, secure, or safe atmosphere for the family.

   _____

   _____

4. **T** **F** You should try to develop positive relationships with all family members.

   _____

   _____

5. **T** **F** You should punish the misbehaving child the way the parents would.

   _____

   _____

6. **T** **F** Bedtime rituals should be eliminated if the child is ill.

   _____

   _____

7. **T** **F** Sudden departure of a caregiver should be reported immediately.

   _____

   _____

8. **T** **F** Touching the child to provide comfort should depend on the child's culture.

   _____

   _____

FILL-IN-THE-BLANKS

9. How can you help to prevent injuries in infants and children when using the following items?

   a. Baby walker _____

      _____

   b. High chair _____

      _____

   c. Cribs _____

      _____

   d. Electrical appliances, equipment _____

      _____

   e. Strings, cords _____

      _____

   f. Medications, cleaners _____

      _____

   g. Clothing _____

      _____

10. List ways to prevent children from drowning in or around the home. (Do not include pools, spas, whirlpools, and hot tubs.)

a. _____

b. _____

c. _____

11. What safety measures can prevent burns in children?

a. _____

b. _____

c. _____

d. _____

e. _____

f. _____

g. _____

h. _____

i. _____

j. _____

12. What measures can help to prevent poisoning in children?

a. _____

b. _____

c. _____

d. _____

e. _____

f. _____

g. _____

h. _____

i. _____

j. _____

13. Children are at special risk for suffocation. What safety measures can be used to prevent suffocation in infants and children?

a. _____

b. _____

c. _____

d. _____

e. _____

f. _____

g. _____

h. _____

i. _____

j. _____

MULTIPLE CHOICE

Circle the correct answer.

14. Children are vaccinated to _____ certain contagious infections.
    a. prevent catching
    b. cure them of
    c. cause mutation of the pathogens that cause
    d. infect them with

15. Which of the following statements about vaccinating children is true?
    a. If vaccinations were to be discontinued, the rate of disease would go down.
    b. Children need to be vaccinated against viral meningitis.
    c. Vaccines can be given to infants only.
    d. Vaccinations prevent the spread of a certain variety of pathogens.

16. As a general rule of thumb, children should stay home from school or day care if:
    a. they drink normally but pick at their food.
    b. they have a temperature of 37.5°C (99.5°F) and sleep soundly at night.
    c. they have a temperature over 38°C (100.4°F), diarrhea, and vomiting.
    d. they have been on antibiotics for 36 hours.

17. Reyes syndrome is:
    a. a rare congenital condition caused by nuclear radiation.
    b. a rare but often fatal illness linked to taking aspirin to treat influenza or chickenpox.
    c. a condition caused by an allergy to acetaminophen (Tylenol).
    d. a common congenital condition caused by drinking alcohol while pregnant.

18. One of the five most common reasons why children stay home from school or day care is because they:
    a. have chickenpox.
    b. ate too many hot dogs at a birthday party.
    c. have test anxiety.
    d. have conjunctivitis.

19. One of the main principles in supporting challenging children is to:
    a. let them have their way so they can be happy.
    b. encourage and reinforce good behaviours.
    c. yell at them to let them know who is the boss.
    d. never give in to their demands.

MATCHING

Match the safety measure used with the correct risk factor.

20. _____ Never store cleaning products in easy-to-reach areas.

21. _____ Teach children not to eat unknown foods, leaves, stems, seeds, berries, nuts, or bark.

22. _____ Measure the temperature of bath water.

23. _____ Keep one hand on a child lying on a table if you must look away.

24. _____ Do not prop up a baby bottle with a rolled-up towel or blanket.

25. _____ Never leave children unattended in a bathtub.

26. _____ Store cleaners, medicines, and hazardous substances in their original containers.

27. _____ Turn pot and pan handles so they point inward from the front of the stove.

28. _____ Keep cords for drapes, blinds, and shades out of reach of children.

a. Burns

b. Suffocation

c. Falls

d. Poisoning

TRUE OR FALSE

Circle T if the statement promotes a client's sexuality and F if it does not. Rewrite all false statements to make them true.

1. **T**   **F**   Encourage the client to wear a hospital gown at all times.

   _____

   _____

2. **T**   **F**   Protect the client's right to privacy.

   _____

   _____

3. **T**   **F**   Encourage the client to get counselling if the client's sexual attitudes are different from yours.

   _____

   _____

4. **T**   **F**   Knock before you enter a room.

   _____

   _____

5. **T**   **F**   Allow older clients the right to be sexual.

   _____

   _____

6. **T**   **F**   Discourage single older clients from developing new relationships.

   _____

   _____

7. **T**   **F**   Allow couples in the long-term care facility to share the same room.

   _____

   _____

8. **T**   **F**   Discourage a woman from shaving her underarms and legs.

   _____

   _____

FILL-IN-THE-BLANKS

9. What are two common causes of loneliness in the older client?

   a. _____

   b. _____

10. What happens to the roles of children and parents as parents age?

    _____

11. What are some ways loneliness in older people can be prevented?

    a. _____

    b. _____

    c. _____

12. Why are there usually more widows than widowers?

    _____

13. When a partner dies, how is the other partner affected?

    a. Serious _____

    _____ and _____
    problems may occur.

    b. May lose _____

    _____ or attempt

    _____ .

14. Why do older clients who speak a foreign language often have greater loneliness and isolation than others?
    a. Relatives and friends who share cultural

    values may _____ .

    b. Client may not have anyone _____

    _____ and may not

    _____ .

15. How do these physical changes affect the safety of the older person?

    a. Skin is fragile and easily injured _____

    _____ .

    b. Fewer nerve endings _____

    _____ .

    c. Decreasing strength and muscle atrophy

    _____ .

    d. Bones become brittle _____

    _____ .

    e. Reduced sense of touch and pain

    _____ .

    f. Reduced blood flow to brain, loss of

    brain cells _____

    _____ .

16. Older clients often complain of feeling cold. What are some ways you can safely provide warmth?

    a. _____

    b. _____

    c. _____

17. How can loss of bone and muscle strength be slowed?

    a. _____

    b. _____

18. Touch and sensitivity to _____

    _____ and _____

    _____ are reduced with aging.

19. What body system will be affected by the care measures described?
    a. Performing range-of-motion exercises

    _____

    b. Providing a sweater and a lap blanket for

    a client who is cold _____

    _____

    c. Allowing the older client to rest or nap

    more during the day _____

    _____

    d. Placing the client in a semi-Fowler's

    position _____

    _____

20. What types of food should older adults avoid?

    _____

21. Urine may be more concentrated because of

_____ and

_____ .

22. Urinary frequency or urgency may occur

because _____

_____ weaken and

_____ decreases.

23. Men may have _____

or _____
because of prostate gland enlargement.

24. The support worker can help the client at
risk for urinary tract infections by providing

_____ .

25. Why should you encourage an older client to
reduce fluid intake after 5:00 P.M.?

_____

26. How can the support worker promote
normal breathing in the older client?

a. _____

b. _____

c. _____

27. What are some ways that an older adult may
express closeness and intimacy without
having intercourse?

a. _____

b. _____

c. _____

d. _____

MULTIPLE CHOICE

Circle the correct answer.

28. Which of these statements describes sexuality?
    a. It involves the whole personality and the
       body.
    b. It is not influenced by social, cultural,
       and spiritual factors.
    c. It is not present from birth.
    d. It is not done for pleasure or to produce
       children.

29. Which of these statements is true about
    sexuality and the older adult?
    a. After menopause, women are no longer
       interested in having sexual relations.
    b. A man cannot have an erection as he gets
       older.
    c. Sexual relationships are psychologically
       and physically important to the older
       adult.
    d. Orgasm may be less intense and longer
       in duration.

30. Which of the following physical changes is
    most likely to cause confusion or behavioural
    changes in an older client?
    a. Respiratory infections
    b. Lack of exercise
    c. Blood flow to the brain is reduced
    d. Poor fluid intake

31. Why does an older client usually require a
    bath only twice a week?
    a. Less exercise is done, so frequent bathing
       is unnecessary.
    b. Fewer baths decrease the possibility of
       injury from falls in the tub.
    c. Skin becomes drier with aging and is
       easily damaged by frequent bathing.
    d. Muscles atrophy and strength is reduced.

32. Why should you avoid applying heat to the feet of an older client?
    a. The skin is dry and has decreased oil glands.
    b. More fold lines and wrinkles appear in the skin.
    c. The feet may become infected more easily.
    d. Decreased sensitivity to heat may increase the risk of burns.

33. Older adults often complain that food has no taste. This happens because:
    a. memory is shorter in older adults.
    b. the number of taste buds decreases with aging.
    c. the ability to feel heat and cold decreases.
    d. a progressive loss of brain cells occurs.

MATCHING

Match the examples given with the benefits of working or retiring and the negative aspects of retirement.

34. _____ Time to travel

35. _____ More leisure time

36. _____ Poor health and aging

37. _____ Increased medical bills with less income

38. _____ Personal fulfillment and usefulness

39. _____ Friendship formed with co-workers

40. _____ Reduced income forces lifestyle changes

41. _____ Time to do as you wish

42. _____ Meets basic needs of love and belonging and self-esteem

43. _____ Reward for lifetime of work

a. Benefit of retirement

b. Negative aspect of retirement

c. Benefit of working

Match the effects of aging with the correct type of change. Some may have more than one answer.

44. _____ Greying hair

45. _____ Preparing for one's own death

46. _____ Death of a partner

47. _____ Slower movements

48. _____ Retirement

a. Physical

b. Psychological

c. Social

DIAGRAMS

63. Identify the parts of the hands that are frequently missed during handwashing.

64. Identify the part of the gown that is considered contaminated after use.

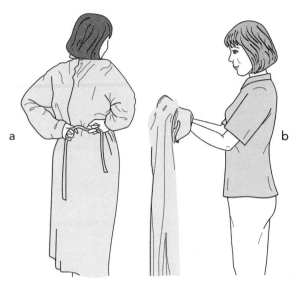

a   b

65. Identify the part of the sterile field that is considered contaminated.

TRUE OR FALSE

Circle T for true or F for false. Rewrite all false statements to make them true.

1. T   F   Usually, the time between abusive events gradually shortens.

    _____

    _____

2. T   F   More women are abused by spouses than men.

    _____

    _____

3. T   F   People who are abused often deny the abuse.

    _____

    _____

4. T   F   Slapping a child is not considered abuse.

    _____

    _____

5. T   F   Emotional and physical abuse are the most common types of abuse of older adults.

    _____

    _____

6. T   F   Ageism is another cause of abuse.

    _____

    _____

7. T   F   Failing to provide privacy is not a form of abuse.

    _____

    _____

8. T   F   Changes in mental function can cause someone to become sexually abusive.

    _____

    _____

9. T   F   Masturbation may be the result of urinary problems in a confused client.

    _____

    _____

10. T   F   The best way to handle client who is masturbating in public is to tell the client to stop.

    _____

    _____

11. T   F   You are legally responsible to report child abuse and (in some jurisdictions) abuse within facilities.

    _____

    _____

12. T   F   Sexual harassment is not considered sexual abuse.

    _____

    _____

13. **T   F**   Abuse is usually triggered by an event related to the victim.

_____

_____

14. **T   F**   People who were abused as children are not likely to abuse their own children because they know what it was like.

_____

_____

15. **T   F**   In most provinces, you do not have to report abuse of older adults to a public authority if it occurs in home care settings.

_____

_____

FILL-IN-THE-BLANKS

16. The three phases in the cycle of abuse are:

a. _____ .

b. _____ .

c. _____ .

17. A person is more likely to be abusive if he or she:

a. _____ .

b. _____ .

c. _____ .

d. _____ .

18. Certain situations increase the risk of child abuse. They are:

a. _____ .

b. _____ .

c. _____ .

d. _____ .

19. Why do abused older adults choose not to complain about the abuse?

a. _____

b. _____

c. _____

d. _____

20. Examples of how workers might abuse clients in a facility or home are:

a. _____ .

b. _____ .

c. _____ .

d. _____ .

e. _____ .

f. _____ .

21. What are some examples of abuse that a support worker may encounter from clients?

a. _____

b. _____

c. _____

d. _____

e. _____

22. What can you do when a client is being abusive?

   a. _____

   b. _____

   c. _____

   d. _____

   e. _____

   f. _____

23. Give three signs or symptoms of each type of abuse.

   Physical abuse

   a. _____

   b. _____

   c. _____

   Sexual abuse

   a. _____

   b. _____

   c. _____

   Emotional abuse

   a. _____

   b. _____

   c. _____

   Financial abuse

   a. _____

   b. _____

   c. _____

Neglect

   a. _____

   b. _____

   c. _____

24. What should you do if a client tells you that he or she is being abused?

   a. _____

   b. _____

   c. _____

   d. _____

   e. _____

MULTIPLE CHOICE

Circle the correct answer.

25. If you suspect a client is being abused, you should:
   a. call the police.
   b. talk to the family.
   c. report it to the nurse.
   d. talk to the client being abused.

26. If you are dealing with an agitated or aggressive client, which of these measures would be most helpful?
   a. Talk to the client in a calm manner.
   b. Place your hand on the client's arm to prevent injury.
   c. Close the door so that other people are not upset.
   d. Promise the client you will not tell anyone else about his or her behaviour.

27. During the "honeymoon phase" of the cycle of abuse:
    a. the abuser begins to get moodier and stressed.
    b. the abuse can escalate easily even if unprovoked.
    c. the abuser often blames the victim for the abuse.
    d. the abuser is very apologetic for what happened.

28. Mrs. Jones is not allowed to go to the bank. Her son insists in handling all of her finances. This is an example of:
    a. neglect.
    b. physical abuse.
    c. financial abuse.
    d. sexual abuse.

29. Mrs. Jones's son insists on changing her incontinence briefs. This might be a sign of:
    a. neglect.
    b. physical abuse.
    c. financial abuse.
    d. sexual abuse.

30. Mrs. Jones cannot speak English. Her son refuses to translate things for her, especially legal documents, such as the deed to her house. This might be a sign of:
    a. neglect.
    b. physical abuse.
    c. financial abuse.
    d. sexual abuse.

31. You are meeting your client, Mrs. Yil, for the first time in her home. While talking to her, you notice that she is very groggy. What should you do?
    a. Try to wake her up.
    b. Notify your supervisor to ask what to do.
    c. Look in her cupboards for medication bottles or empty bottles of alcohol.
    d. Ask her if you should come back another time when she is more awake.

32. You have been supporting Mrs. Yil for several weeks. During that time, you have noticed that Mrs. Yil is very quiet whenever her daughter comes to visit her. You suspect abuse but cannot prove it. What should you do?
    a. Ask Mrs. Yil after her daughter leaves.
    b. Ask Mrs. Yil's daughter if she has noticed how quiet her mother is.
    c. Telephone the police and make a complaint.
    d. Discuss this situation with your supervisor.

33. Miss Keys scratches and punches when it is time for her shower. What should you do?
    a. Stay calm and protect yourself.
    b. Refuse to bathe Mrs. Keys.
    c. Use silence and ignore her behaviour.
    d. Report her behaviour to the nurse in charge.

34. When a client is angry and demanding, it is important to:
    a. ask the nurse to talk to the client.
    b. ignore the client until her behaviour improves.
    c. treat the person with respect and dignity.
    d. tell the client how irritating she is to the staff.

35. A term used to describe infants, babies, or children who are below the norms for body weight, growth, or cognitive development is:
    a. neglected.
    b. failure to thrive.
    c. refusal to grow.
    d. idiopathic weight challenge.

MATCHING

Match the correct terms with their definitions.

36. _____ Failure to meet basic needs

37. _____ Misuse of a client's money

38. _____ Force or violence that causes injury

39. _____ Unwanted sexual activity

40. _____ Words or actions that inflict mental harm

a. Sexual abuse

b. Physical abuse

c. Emotional abuse

d. Financial abuse

e. Neglect

Match the different forms of client abuse with the appropriate description.

41. _____ Threatening punishment or deprival of needs

42. _____ Inflicting punishment on the body

43. _____ Harassing or attacking a client sexually

44. _____ Client's money is used by another person without consent

45. _____ Providing care against the client's wishes

a. Physical

b. Violation of rights

c. Sexual

d. Financial

e. Emotional

46. Name the types of child abuse described in the examples below.

A welt in the shape of a belt buckle is found on the body.

a. _____

A child is kissed, touched, or fondled inappropriately.

b. _____

A child is deprived of food and clothing.

c. _____

A child is forced to engage in sexual activity for money.

d. _____

A child's need for affection and attention is not met.

e. _____

A child is threatened and called names.

f. _____

Promoting Client Well-Being

TRUE OR FALSE

Circle T for true or F for false. Rewrite all false statements to make them true.

1. **T**   **F**   Personal items in a client's unit are arranged as the individual prefers.

    _____

    _____

2. **T**   **F**   The support worker may throw away any items in the client's unit that are in the way.

    _____

    _____

3. **T**   **F**   Make sure the client can reach the telephone, television, and light controls.

    _____

    _____

4. **T**   **F**   Moving furniture or belongings may be a safety hazard for a client with poor vision.

    _____

    _____

5. **T**   **F**   Distraction involves creating an image in the mind.

    _____

    _____

FILL-IN-THE-BLANKS

6. If a client complains of pain, the client

    _____ .

7. What type of pain is felt suddenly from injury, disease, trauma, or surgery?

    _____

8. How do these factors affect pain?

    a. Past experience

    _____

    b. Anxiety

    _____

    c. Rest and sleep

    _____

    d. Attention

    _____

    e. Value or meaning of pain

    _____

    f. Support from others

    _____

    g. Culture

    _____

    h. Age

    _____

9. The nurse needs certain information to assess the client's pain. What questions could you ask to help gather this information for the nurse?

    a. Location _____

        _____

    b. Onset and duration _____

        _____

    c. Intensity _____

        _____

    d. Description _____

        _____

    e. Factors causing pain _____

        _____

    f. Vital signs _____

        _____

    g. Other signs and symptoms _____

        _____

10. What reaction to pain may occur with a client from these cultures?

    a. Philippines _____

        _____

    b. Vietnam _____

        _____

    c. China _____

        _____

11. Why are older clients at greater risk for undetected disease or injury?

    _____

12. What body responses may be signs and symptoms of pain?

    a. _____

    b. _____

    c. _____

    d. _____

    e. _____

13. What are some of the safety measures used when the client is receiving strong pain medications?

    a. _____

    b. _____

    c. _____

    d. _____

14. How long should you wait to perform procedures after pain medications are given?

    _____

15. The nurse asks you to assist with these measures to control pain. What is done with each one?

    a. Distraction _____

        _____

    b. Relaxation _____

        _____

    c. Guided imagery _____

        _____

16. When a client experiences pain, it cannot be seen, heard, felt, or smelled. How can you know the client has pain?

    _____

LABELLING

20. Name each piece of linen on the bed.

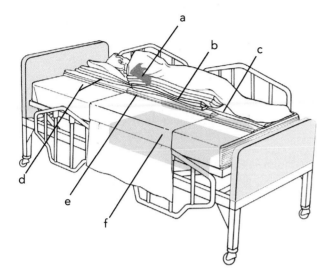

a. _____

b. _____

c. _____

d. _____

e. _____

f. _____

21. Arrange in order the steps used to make a mitred corner.

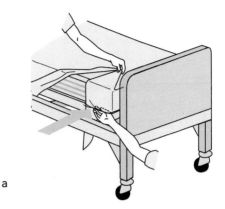

a

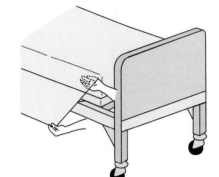

b

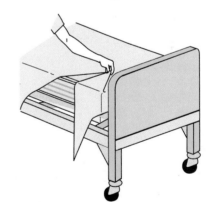

c

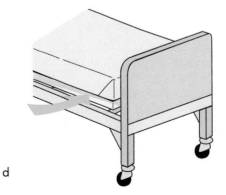

d

LINEN SCRAMBLE

22. You are getting ready to change bed linens.
Number the linens you collect in the correct
order from 1 to 9.

_____ Bedspread

_____ Plastic drawsheet

_____ Bottom sheet

_____ Bath blanket

_____ Cotton drawsheet

_____ Mattress pad

_____ Top sheet

_____ Pillowcases

_____ Blanket

TRUE OR FALSE

Circle T for true or F for false. Rewrite all false statements to make them true.

1. **T   F**   The body becomes swollen if too much sugar is retained.

    _____

    _____

2. **T   F**   When a healthy client eats more sodium than the body needs, it will be excreted.

    _____

    _____

3. **T   F**   A client with diabetes will retain salt in the body.

    _____

    _____

4. **T   F**   A "moderate sodium-restricted diet" allows the client to eat pickles and olives.

    _____

    _____

5. **T   F**   When a client has diabetes, sugar builds up in the bloodstream.

    _____

    _____

6. **T   F**   When a client is placed on a diabetic diet, only three meals each day are allowed.

    _____

    _____

7. **T   F**   A diet that allows water, gelatin, and popsicles would be a clear liquid diet.

    _____

    _____

8. **T   F**   A client who has constipation may be helped by a high-fibre diet.

    _____

    _____

9. **T   F**   Many special diets involve between-meal nourishments such as crackers and milk.

    _____

    _____

FILL-IN-THE-BLANKS

10. Convert the following amounts into cubic centimetres (cc) or millilitres (mL) using this scale.

    1 oz = 30 cc (mL)
    1 cup = 240 cc (mL)
    1 quart = 1000 cc (mL)

    a. 6-oz cup of coffee =

        _____

    b. 8 oz of milk =

        _____

    c. 1 quart of water =

        _____

    d. 2 cups of tea =

        _____

e. 4 oz of gelatin =

_____

f. 5 oz of orange juice =

_____

g. 12 oz of broth =

_____

h. half-cup of sherbet =

_____

11. How many calories are in:

a. 1 g of carbohydrate?

_____

b. 1 g of fat?

_____

c. 1 g of protein?

_____

12. Chopped foods may be added to an infant's

diet at about _____ of age.

13. What dietary guidelines are recommended
for healthy eating?

a. _____

b. _____

c. _____

d. _____

e. _____

14. How large is one serving of meat, poultry, or

fish? _____

How many servings of meat, poultry, or fish

are recommended daily? _____

15. In what country is beef generally not eaten?

_____

16. What would be the best way you could help
to prepare these clients to eat?

a. Client who must stay in bed

_____

b. Client who is allowed out of bed

_____

17. In what ways, other than positioning, can
you assist a client to get ready for meals?

a. _____

b. _____

c. _____

d. _____

e. _____

f. _____

18. How do these physical changes affect the
older client's appetite or food intake?

a. Decrease in saliva

_____

b. Taste and smell dull

_____

c. Secretion of digestive juices decreases

_____

d. Loss of teeth and ill-fitting dentures

_____

e. Decreased peristalsis

_____

19. If an older client must avoid high-fibre foods, what foods may be eaten to prevent constipation?

_____

20. Why are the following actions important for safety and comfort when feeding a client?

a. Provide a relaxed mood

_____

b. Provide time and privacy to pray

_____

c. Use spoon to feed

_____

d. Offer small portions (spoon that is one-third teaspoon full)

_____

e. Offer fluids during meal

_____

f. Engage in conversation

_____

g. Sit so you face client

_____

h. Encourage client to feed himself or herself

_____

21. What type of special diet would be ordered for the following situations?

a. First diet after surgery

_____

b. Constipation and colon disorders

_____

c. Weight gain and certain thyroid imbalances

_____

d. Heart disease, gallbladder disease

_____

e. Burns, high fever, infection

_____

22. If there is too much sodium in the diet, the body retains more _____ _____. This increases the workload on the _____ _____ .

23. On a sodium-restricted diet, what is the only food group that has no restrictions?

_____

24. The client with diabetes must eat at regular times to maintain _____ _____ .

25. When a client has dysphagia, what is done to the food to meet the client's needs?

_____

26. What are six common causes of dehydration?

a. _____

b. _____

c. _____

d. _____

e. _____

f. _____

27. How much water does an adult need each day to survive?

    _____

28. How much fluid is needed each day to maintain normal fluid balance?

    _____

29. When fluids are restricted, why is frequent oral hygiene important?

    _____

30. List the four food groups included in the Food Guide.

    a. _____

    b. _____

    c. _____

    d. _____

31. Identify the food group to which each of the following items belong.

    a. Crackers _____

    b. Kidney beans _____

    c. Potatoes _____

    d. Pineapple chunks _____

    e. Peanut butter _____

    f. Ice milk _____

    g. Chocolate bar _____

    h. Oatmeal _____

    i. Carrots _____

    j. Sour cream _____

32. Should an older client increase or decrease these dietary elements? Why or when?

    a. Calories _____

       Why? _____

    b. Fluids _____

       Why? _____

    c. Protein _____

       Why? _____

    d. Soft bulk _____

       Why? _____

    e. Fried, fatty foods _____

       Why? _____

MULTIPLE CHOICE

Circle the correct answer.

33. Why are carbohydrates important in the diet?
    a. Supply products for tissue growth and repair
    b. Provide energy and bulk for bowel elimination
    c. Provide energy and flavour
    d. Supply vitamins that are needed daily

34. What can you give a client who has an order for NPO?
    a. Unlimited fluids
    b. No food or fluids
    c. Small amounts of fluids
    d. Only clear liquids

35. What effect may cultural and religious beliefs have on nutrition?
    a. Certain types of food may be restricted.
    b. Method of preparation may be part of beliefs.
    c. Certain foods are eaten and others are avoided.
    d. All of the above may be part of beliefs.

36. Which of these foods would not be included as liquid intake?
    a. Tomato soup
    b. Cream of wheat cereal
    c. Beef vegetable soup
    d. Chocolate pudding

37. Which of the following statements describes assistive dining?
    a. One client is fed by one support worker to reduce stimulation.
    b. Food is placed on platters or dishes and the clients serve themselves.
    c. Clients are served food at the table as in a restaurant.
    d. Four clients are seated at the horseshoe-shaped table and are fed by one support worker.

MATCHING

Match the nutrient with the reason it is important to good health.

38. _____ Needed for tooth and bone formation

39. _____ Tissue growth and repair

40. _____ Provides energy and adds flavour

41. _____ Provides energy and fibre for elimination

42. _____ Does not provide calories but is needed for certain body functions

a. Protein

b. Carbohydrates

c. Fats

d. Vitamins

e. Minerals

Match the vitamin with its major function.

43. _____ Healthy eyes, healthy skin and mucous membranes, protein and carbohydrate metabolism

44. _____ Formation of substances that hold tissues together

45. _____ Formation of red blood cells, nervous system functioning

46. _____ Blood clotting

47. _____ Normal reproduction

48. _____ Growth, vision, healthy hair and skin

49. _____ Muscle tone, nerve function, digestion

50. _____ Protein, fat, and carbohydrate metabolism

51. _____ Formation of red blood cells, functioning of intestine

52. _____ Absorption and metabolism of calcium and phosphorus, healthy bones

a. Vitamin A

b. Thiamine

c. Riboflavin

d. Niacin

e. Vitamin B_{12}

f. Folic acid

g. Ascorbic acid

h. Vitamin D

i. Vitamin E

j. Vitamin K

Match the mineral with its major function.

53. _____ Formation of bone and teeth, nerve and muscle function

54. _____ Thyroid gland function

55. _____ Fluid balance

56. _____ Formation of bone and teeth, blood clotting

57. _____ Allows red blood cells to carry oxygen

58. _____ Nerve function, heart function

a. Calcium

b. Phosphorus

c. Iron

d. Iodine

e. Sodium

f. Potassium

LABELLING

59. Label the plate with numbers so that you can describe the location of food to a blind client.
   a. Where would you tell the blind client to find the meat?

   _____

   b. Where would you tell the blind client to find the baked potato?

   _____

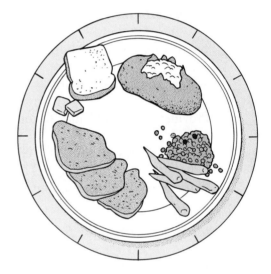

33 Rehabilitation Care

TRUE OR FALSE

Circle T for true or F for false. Rewrite all false statements to make them true.

1. **T   F**   A disability does not affect the client's psychological well-being. It is only a physical problem.

   _____

   _____

2. **T   F**   Rehabilitation begins by preventing complications.

   _____

   _____

3. **T   F**   Rehabilitation often takes less time in older clients than in other age groups.

   _____

   _____

4. **T   F**   Health care workers as well as the client and family members are part of the rehabilitation team.

   _____

   _____

5. **T   F**   When the health care team sets goals for the client, they can never be changed.

   _____

   _____

FILL-IN-THE-BLANKS

6. The following goals of rehabilitation are common:

   a. _____

   b. _____

   c. _____

   d. _____

7. The goal of a prosthesis is

   _____ .

8. Examples of orthoses are:

   a. _____

   b. _____

   c. _____

   d. _____

9. Rehabilitation can occur in different settings. List some of the settings.

   a. _____

   b. _____

   c. _____

   d. _____

10. Common health problems requiring rehabilitation are:

   a. _____

   b. _____

c. _____

d. _____

e. _____

f. _____

g. _____

h. _____

11. Why is good skin care important in rehabilitation?

_____

12. How can an electric toothbrush help a client with a disability become more independent?

_____

_____

13. How can you improve the quality of life for a client with a disability?

a. Right to privacy

_____

b. Preferences

_____

c. Dignity

_____

d. Safety

_____

e. Independence

_____

MATCHING

Match the following words with the correct definitions.

20. _____ Process of restoring a person to the highest possible level of function

21. _____ Self-care activities performed to remain independent

22. _____ Helps a person regain health and strength

14. Why is the home assessed by the rehabilitation team before a client goes home?

_____

MULTIPLE CHOICE

Circle the correct answer.

15. An orthotic is:
    a. an artificial replacement for missing body parts.
    b. the process of correcting a deformity.
    c. an apparatus worn for support.
    d. the process of restoring a client to the highest level of functioning possible.

16. Rehabilitation:
    a. is often slow and frustrating.
    b. occurs quickly.
    c. is carried out only in a hospital.
    d. does not involve the family.

17. Occupational therapists on the rehabilitation team:
    a. lead and coordinate rehabilitation.
    b. assess the performance of activities of daily living.
    c. test speech.
    d. coordinate home care.

18. Social workers on the rehabilitation team:
    a. provide counselling.
    b. help with physical therapy.
    c. coordinate and provide care at every stage.
    d. evaluate strength.

19. The goals of rehabilitation are:
    a. to restore function to former levels.
    b. to improve functional abilities.
    c. to learn new skills.
    d. all of the above.

a. Activities of daily living

b. Independence

c. Rehabilitation

TRUE OR FALSE

Circle T for true or F for false. Rewrite all false statements to make them true.

1. **T** **F** Aggression follows a progressive cycle even though it seems to happen suddenly.

   _____

   _____

2. **T** **F** Depression is a type of dementia that is rarely cured.

   _____

   _____

3. **T** **F** Aggressive clients should be restrained.

   _____

   _____

4. **T** **F** Anxiety is displayed in all mental health disorders.

   _____

   _____

5. **T** **F** Only illegal drugs are abused.

   _____

   _____

6. **T** **F** Communication is important when caring for persons with mental health disorders.

   _____

   _____

7. **T** **F** Panic is the highest level of anxiety.

   _____

   _____

8. **T** **F** A panic attack occurs suddenly with no obvious reason.

   _____

   _____

9. **T** **F** When a panic attack occurs, the client may experience chest pain.

   _____

   _____

10. **T** **F** A phobia involves intense fear of an object or situation.

    _____

    _____

11. **T** **F** Depression is at one extreme of the bipolar disorders.

    _____

    _____

12. **T** **F** In the manic phase, the person feels worthless.

    _____

    _____

13. **T** **F** Depression in the older adult is rarely overlooked.

    _____

    _____

14. **T   F**   Major depression can occur at any age.

_____

_____

15. **T   F**   Psychosis is a mental disorder in which the perception of reality is impaired.

_____

_____

16. **T   F**   Delusion is a form of hallucination.

_____

_____

17. **T   F**   The term *hallucinations* refers to strange beliefs.

_____

_____

18. **T   F**   Schizophrenia affects one's ability to function in all aspects of life.

_____

_____

19. **T   F**   Someone who has schizophrenia has a split personality.

_____

_____

20. **T   F**   The person who has schizophrenia has problems knowing what is real and what is not.

_____

_____

21. **T   F**   Paranoid clients may have a great many religious delusions.

_____

FILL-IN-THE-BLANKS

22. What are some of the causes of mental health disorders?

a. _____

b. _____

c. _____

d. _____

23. The various forms of psychotherapy include:

a. _____ .

b. _____ .

c. _____ .

d. _____ .

24. A person suffering from schizophrenia may exhibit the following behaviours:

a. _____

b. _____

c. _____

d. _____

25. Signs and symptoms of depression include:

a. _____ .

b. _____ .

c. _____ .

d. _____ .

26. An obsession is a

_____ .

27. A compulsion is

_____ .

28. Why does a person act on an obsessive idea?

_____

29. If a person believes he or she is the prime minister of Canada, what type of false belief is present?

_____

30. What are the two most common extremes of a bipolar disorder?

_____

31. An older client has the following symptoms: fatigue, slow or unreliable memory, agitation, and thoughts of death. It may be that the person is suffering from

_____ .

32. A client with _____ craves food. After eating, the person induces

_____ .

33. Why does a person with bulimia take diuretics?

_____

_____

34. What are the following statements describing?
   • Thinking and behaviour are disturbed
   • Delusions and hallucinations are present
   • Difficulty relating to others and the world

_____

35. What are the following statements describing?
   • Vague, uneasy feelings
   • Feels sense of danger or harm
   • Occurs in response to stress
   • Unaware of source of uneasy feeling

_____

36. What are the following statements describing?
   • Has extreme mood swings
   • At times feels very sad, lonely, worthless
   • Tends to run in families
   • At times has much energy and is excited

_____

37. What are the following statements describing?
   • Abusive
   • Paranoid
   • Distrusts others
   • Irresponsible

_____

MULTIPLE CHOICE

Circle the correct answer.

38. Which of these may cause mental health disorders?
   a. Inability to cope with stress
   b. Chemical imbalances in the body
   c. Characteristics inherited from parents
   d. All of the above

39. Which of the following is an example of an unhealthy coping mechanism?
   a. Going for a walk
   b. Exercising
   c. Chain smoking
   d. Having a piece of cake with a meal

40. An older adult may not be diagnosed with depression because:
   a. it rarely occurs in an older adult.
   b. treatment of physical problems is more important in the older adult.
   c. the older person may be thought to have dementia.
   d. it is usually mild and does not require treatment.

41. Which of these would be present if the person has delusions of persecution?
    a. Seeing, hearing, or feeling something that is not there
    b. Not sleeping or taking time to tend to self-care needs
    c. Believing that one is mistreated, abused, or harassed
    d. Having poor judgement and morals and lacking ethics

42. When a girl has anorexia nervosa, which of these behaviours is she likely to display?
    a. Diets even though she becomes emaciated
    b. Withdraws from the world and shows no interest in others
    c. Retreats to behaviours of a younger-aged child
    d. Has delusions or hallucinations

43. Which of these substances can be abused?
    a. Legal drugs
    b. Illegal drugs
    c. Alcohol
    d. All of the above

44. Which of the following statements about mental health disorders is true?
    a. Defence mechanisms are a symptom of mental illness.
    b. Persons with paranoid personality disorders trust others.
    c. Depression disorders are common in adults only.
    d. Bipolar disorders are characterized by extreme mood swings.

45. What is the best response to use when caring for a depressed client?
    a. "Let me tell you a funny story."
    b. "Would you like to talk about it?"
    c. "Cheer up and don't look so sad."
    d. "Don't worry. Everything will be all right."

46. Your client Mr. White has extreme suspiciousness of others and experiences hallucinations. Which approach by the staff would be the most threatening to Mr. White?
    a. Forthright and honest
    b. Friendly and emotionally detached
    c. Warm and nurturing
    d. Tolerant and reserved

47. Mr. White becomes very angry and states that someone has been in his room and has taken his razor. He is swearing and yelling at the staff. Your best response is:
    a. "I don't blame you for being angry."
    b. "That doesn't make any sense. I don't know who would want your razor."
    c. to say nothing but begin to look in his bedside unit.
    d. "This is very upsetting. Can you show me where you usually keep your razor?"

48. Which statement with regard to suicide is correct?
    a. Suicidal intent is a sign of a serious physical health problem.
    b. More women commit suicide than men.
    c. Men use less violent means to commit suicide.
    d. Suicide is a common cause of death among adolescents.

49. Which is a common warning signal for suicidal intent?
    a. Giving away prized possessions
    b. Extreme suspiciousness
    c. Extreme interest in a dangerous sport
    d. Performing well in school

50. When working with clients who have a distorted perception of reality, the support worker will generally be most effective if he or she:
    a. encourages the client to discuss the voices they hear.
    b. tries to reorient the client back to reality.
    c. avoids all unnecessary physical contact.
    d. changes the subject matter.

TRUE OR FALSE

Circle T for true or F for false. Rewrite all false statements to make them true.

1. **T F** Only tell a confused client the date and time once a day.

   _____

   _____

2. **T F** When caring for confused clients, you should provide newspapers and magazines and access to television and radio.

   _____

   _____

3. **T F** It is all right to re-arrange the furniture or the belongings of a confused client.

   _____

   _____

4. **T F** Delirium is a permanent, chronic mental confusion.

   _____

   _____

5. **T F** Delirium is an emergency.

   _____

   _____

6. **T F** Repetitious behaviour is usually harmless, and the client can be allowed to continue with the actions.

   _____

   _____

7. **T F** People with Alzheimer's disease can control their behaviours of forgetfulness, incontinence, agitation, or rudeness if they are shown how.

   _____

   _____

8. **T F** Alzheimer's disease progresses slowly at a predictable rate in all people.

   _____

   _____

9. **T F** It is important to reason with the cognitively impaired client as a first step when the client is angry and aggressive.

   _____

   _____

10. **T F** Considering the behaviour of individuals who have mental illness and cognitive impairment, they are not likely candidates for abuse.

   _____

   _____

11. **T F** As a caregiver of clients with cognitive impairment, when entering their personal space, it is important that you approach in an assertive, controlling manner.

   _____

   _____

FILL-IN-THE-BLANKS

12. What are the early warning signs of dementia?

    a. _____

    b. _____

    c. _____

    d. _____

    e. _____

    f. _____

    g. _____

13. Delirium is common in _____ with _____ illnesses.

14. The risk of Alzheimer's disease increases after the age of _____ .

15. Why is a person with dementia in danger of having accidents?

    _____

16. List some of the behaviours associated with early-stage dementia.

    a. _____

    b. _____

    c. _____

    d. _____

    e. _____

    f. _____

    g. _____

    h. _____

17. These are problems that occur with dementia. Describe each one or the behaviour that is displayed with the problem.

    a. Wandering _____

       _____

    b. Sundowning _____

       _____

    c. Hallucinations _____

       _____

    d. Delusions _____

       _____

    e. Catastrophic reaction _____

       _____

    f. Agitation and restlessness _____

       _____

    g. Aggression and combativeness _____

       _____

    h. Screaming _____

       _____

    i. Abnormal sexual behaviour _____

       _____

    j. Repetitive behaviours _____

       _____

18. How can a caregiver cause agitation and restlessness?

    _____

19. List ways caregivers help to calm a person with dementia who screams.

    a. _____

    b. _____

    c. _____

    d. _____

    e. _____

20. How can you help a client with Alzheimer's disease who displays abnormal sexual behaviour?

    _____

    _____

21. Why does sundowning occur in a client with Alzheimer's disease?

    a. _____

    b. _____

    c. _____

22. What response may occur if the client with Alzheimer's disease has too much stimulation at one time?

    _____

23. What are reasons why a family usually decides to place a person with Alzheimer's disease in a long-term care facility?

    a. _____

    b. _____

    c. _____

    d. _____

24. Complete these statements that relate to caring for a confused client.

    a. Face the client and _____

       _____ .

    b. Explain what _____

       _____ .

    c. Give short, simple _____

       _____ .

    d. Keep calendars and clocks with _____

       _____ .

    e. Allow the client to place _____

       _____ .

    f. Ask _____

       questions. Allow enough time _____

       _____ .

    g. Maintain _____

       _____ atmosphere.

    h. Remind the client of _____

       _____ .

25. How can you maintain the day–night cycle for a confused client?

    a. _____

    b. _____

    c. _____

26. What can you do to maintain a confused client's routine?

    _____

    Why is this important?

    _____

    _____

27. What is meant by the "sandwich generation?"

    _____

28. Why are locks placed at the top or bottom of a door to prevent wandering?

    _____

29. Why is it ineffective to argue or try to reason with a client with Alzheimer's disease?

    _____

MULTIPLE CHOICE

Circle the correct answer.

30. Which of the following interventions would not help when caring for a client who is confused?
    a. State your name and show your name tag.
    b. Give very detailed answers to questions to help the client understand.
    c. Call the client by name each time you are in contact with him or her.
    d. Encourage the client to wear glasses and a hearing aid if needed.

31. Which of these is helpful when a client with Alzheimer's disease is agitated?
    a. Keep the client in a calm, quiet environment.
    b. Complete care very quickly.
    c. Place the client in a darkened room.
    d. Take the client to an area with music, activity, and people.

32. How can a client who wanders be protected?
    a. Make sure the client receives medication to calm him or her down.
    b. Restrain the client to prevent movement or wandering.
    c. Go with the client who insists on going outside.
    d. Explain to the client why going outside is not possible.

33. Mrs. Burns has Alzheimer's disease. She has been having hallucinations that "kitty cats" are in her closet. What might be helpful?
    a. Distract her by showing her something else.
    b. Explain to her that there are no cats in the facility she lives in.
    c. Ask her to draw a picture of the cat.
    d. Turn up the radio.

34. When a client suffering with Alzheimer's disease says "I want to go home," it may be appropriate to answer:
    a. "The weather outside is beautiful today."
    b. "Home is where you are at the present."
    c. "Tell me about your home."
    d. "Let's go for a walk."

35. A broad term describing a progressive deterioration of intellectual function is known as:
    a. dementia.
    b. mental illness.
    c. senility.
    d. schizophrenia.

36. What guideline should the support worker follow when caring for clients with delirium?
    a. Once clients are on medication, their behaviours will always improve.
    b. It is more important to contain the behaviour rather than restrain behaviour.
    c. Agitated clients should be confronted to assess the problem.
    d. Delirium is never reversible, and the family should be aware of this.

37. When dealing with a client exhibiting aggressive or violent behaviour, the support worker should:
    a. immediately demand that the client sit down.
    b. approach the client alone so he or she does not feel threatened.
    c. distract the client by turning the television on.
    d. remain at arms' length at all times.

38. What is a classic sign of Alzheimer's disease?
  a. Problems finding or speaking the right word
  b. Repeating statements over and over
  c. Engaging in reckless behaviour
  d. Forgetting how to perform long division

39. Mr. Parco has Alzheimer's disease. Which of the following is a sign of this?
  a. Fever
  b. Nausea and vomiting
  c. Cursing or swearing
  d. Alopecia

40. Mr. Jones tends to wander. Which statement about wandering is true?
  a. There is always a cause.
  b. It is always caused by drug side effects.
  c. Stress and anxiety might be the cause.
  d. The client will eventually get bored and will stop on his own.

MATCHING

Match each statement with one of the two disorders given.

41. _____ May get lost in familiar places

42. _____ Can occur after surgery

43. _____ Anger, restlessness, depression, and irritability may occur

44. _____ May be caused by losses of hearing and sight

45. _____ Progressive loss of cognitive and social functions

a. Confusion

b. Dementia

Match the symptom of dementia to the stage when it usually first occurs.

46. _____ Restlessness that increases during evening hours

47. _____ Cannot walk or sit

48. _____ Less outgoing and less interested in things

49. _____ Forgets recent events

50. _____ Does not recognize family members

51. _____ May say the same thing over and over

52. _____ Cannot tell the difference between hot and cold

53. _____ Totally incontinent of urine and feces

54. _____ Disoriented to time and place

55. _____ Cannot communicate

56. _____ Has difficulty following directions

a. Stage 1

b. Stage 2

c. Stage 3

Match the area of concern for people with dementia with a strategy to give care in that area.

57. _____ Follow facility policy for locking doors and windows.   a.   Environment

58. _____ Provide plastic eating and drinking utensils.   b.   Communication

59. _____ Tell the client that you will provide protection from harm.   c.   Safety

60. _____ Give consistent responses.   d.   Wandering

61. _____ Provide for the client's food and fluid needs.   e.   Sundowning

62. _____ Try bathing the client when he or she is calm.   f.   Hallucinations and delusions

63. _____ Play music and show movies from the client's past.

64. _____ Make sure the client wears an ID bracelet at all times.   g.   Basic needs

65. _____ Dim lights and play soft music to help calm the client.

66. _____ Approach the client in a calm, quiet manner.

67. _____ Store personal care items in a safe place.

68. _____ Use touch to calm and reassure the client.

69. _____ Keep personal care items where the client can see them.

70. _____ Do not argue with a client who wants to leave.

71. _____ Have equipment ready for any procedure ahead of time.

72. _____ Remove dangerous appliances and power tools from home.

73. _____ Make sure the client has eaten because hunger can increase restlessness.

Speech and Language Disorders

TRUE OR FALSE

Circle T for true or F for false. Rewrite all false statements to make them true.

1. **T** **F** Most people with dementia have apraxia.

   _____

   _____

2. **T** **F** Some people with aphasia cannot understand the message.

   _____

   _____

3. **T** **F** People with expressive aphasia are not aware of their mistakes when speaking.

   _____

   _____

4. **T** **F** Dysarthria is caused by weakness in the muscles used for speech.

   _____

   _____

5. **T** **F** Relationships between family members are not affected when someone has a speech disorder.

   _____

   _____

6. **T** **F** Shopping and cooking are not affected when someone has a communication problem.

   _____

   _____

7. **T** **F** Because you do not need to spend time on communication, you can take less time giving care to someone who cannot speak.

   _____

   _____

8. **T** **F** It is a help to the client to finish words for him or her.

   _____

   _____

9. **T** **F** Use positive statements rather than negative statements.

   _____

   _____

10. **T** **F** Aphasia is seldom permanent.

    _____

    _____

FILL-IN-THE-BLANKS

11. What can cause speech and language disorders?

    a. _____

    b. _____

    c. _____

    d. _____

    e. _____

12. List the three basic types of aphasia and briefly describe the differences.

a. _____

_____

_____

b. _____

_____

_____

c. _____

_____

_____

13. Apraxia of speech means _____ .

People with this disorder_____

_____ .

14. Dysarthria means _____ .

People with this disorder _____

_____ .

15. What are some of the emotions people with speech and language disorders may experience?

a. _____

b. _____

c. _____

d. _____

16. How do you provide compassionate care to clients who have speech or language disorders?

a. _____

_____

_____

b. _____

_____

_____

c. _____

_____

_____

d. _____

_____

_____

17. Some guidelines to effective communication with clients with speech or language disorders are:

a. _____ .

b. _____ .

c. _____ .

d. _____ .

e. _____ .

f. _____ .

79. Place an X on three ~~...~~
ulcers may form on ~~...~~
Fowler's position.

47. Clients with infected and draining wounds
will require more of which two nutrients?
a. Calcium and iron
b. Protein and vitamin C
c. Potassium and phosphorus
d. Vitamins A and D

TRUE O ~~...~~

Circle T fo ~~...~~
statements

1. **T**

2. **T**

3. **T**   Cyar ~~...~~

a

4. **T**

c

Courtesy Laurel Wiersma-Bryan ~~...~~

81. Identify the stages of ~~...~~

a. Stage _____

_____

b. Stage _____

_____

5. **T**

MATCHING

Match the type of wound with the correct description. Some descriptions may be used more than once.

48. _____ Wound containing large amounts of bacteria

49. _____ Wound that does not heal easily

50. _____ Wound created for therapy

51. _____ Wound resulting from trauma

52. _____ Wound occurring from surgical entry of urinary, reproductive, respiratory, or gastro-intestinal system

53. _____ Wound that is not infected; microbes have not entered wound

54. _____ Dermis, epidermis, and subcutaneous tissue are penetrated; muscle and bone may be involved

55. _____ Wound with high risk of infection

56. _____ Wound in which tissues are injured, but the skin is not broken

57. _____ Skin or mucous membrane is broken

58. _____ Wound in which dermis and epidermis of the skin are broken

a. Chronic wound

b. Clean wound

c. Clean-contaminated wound

d. Closed wound

e. Contaminated wound

f. Dirty (infected) wound

g. Full-thickness wound

h. Intentional wound

i. Open wound

j. Partial-thickness wound

k. Unintentional wound

Match the type of wound drainage with the correct description. Some descriptions may be used more than once.

59. _____ Thin, watery drainage that is blood tinged

60. _____ Thick green, yellow, or brown drainage

61. _____ Bloody drainage

62. _____ Clear, watery fluid

a. Purulent drainage

b. Sanguineous drainage

c. Serosanguineous drainage

d. Serous drainage

Match the stage of a
than once.

63. _____ The skin

64. _____ The skin

65. _____ Drainage

66. _____ The colo

67. _____ Muscle a

68. _____ The skin

69. _____ There ma

70. _____ The expo

Match the phase of w
than once.

71. _____ Tissue ce

72. _____ Scar even

73. _____ Lasts up

74. _____ Blood su

75. _____ Begins ab

76. _____ Loss of fu

LABELLING

77. Place an X on six
ulcers may form c
lateral position.

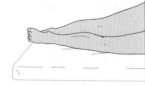

11. What happens to blood vessels and blood
flow when heat is applied for a long time?

_____

12. What people or groups of people are at risk
for burns from heat applications?

a. _____

b. _____

c. _____

d. _____

e. _____

f. _____

g. _____

13. How long may heat or cold be applied?

_____

14. What type of soak is used to clean perineal
or anal wounds?

_____

15. When working in home care, what can be
used to apply ice?

a. _____

b. _____

c. _____

16. How often should you check the skin when
cold compresses are in place?

_____

CROS

Acros

5. Pres
7. Thi
8. Cle
9. Con
   eno
11. Con
13. Thi
14. Acc
    mu
16. Sep
    abd

17. What are the signs of complications when
applying heat or cold?

a. _____

b. _____

c. _____

d. _____

e. _____

f. _____

18. What guidelines should be followed when
you are applying heat or cold?

a. _____

b. _____

c. _____

d. _____

e. _____

f. _____

g. _____

h. _____

i. _____

j. _____

k. _____

l. _____

m. _____

MULTIPLE CHOICE

Circle the correct answer.

19. Which of these factors may make a client more susceptible to burns?
    a. Respiratory disorders
    b. Dehydration
    c. Circulatory disorders
    d. Infections

20. Heat should not be applied to which of these areas?
    a. Metal hip and knee replacements
    b. Joints
    c. Soft tissues
    d. Old fractures

21. A sitz bath may cause the client to feel weak or faint because:
    a. the bath increases pain in the area.
    b. blood flow increases in the pelvic area, and less blood flows to other body parts.
    c. blood flow decreases in the pelvic area, and more blood flows to other body parts.
    d. the client becomes chilled.

22. You applied a commercial cold pack to Jane's ankle as instructed in her care plan. After 3 minutes, she complains of extreme pain to the area. What should you do first?
    a. Check it after another 2 minutes.
    b. Notify your supervisor.
    c. Take her pulse to that area.
    d. Remove the cold pack.

23. Why are people with thin skin at increased risk for burns with heat and cold applications? They:
    a. have better circulation than people with thicker skin.
    b. lack enough of a protective adipose layer.
    c. usually have taken better care of their skin.
    d. lack feeling to their skin.

24. Heat and cold applications must be covered before applying them to a client's skin. Which is the best answer for why this is done?
    a. Protects the heat and cold pads from wear and tear
    b. Keeps the heat and cold pack cleaner and free of germs
    c. Helps to prevent contact burns on the client's skin
    d. Prevents skin irritation from the surface of the pack

MATCHING

Match the types of heat applications with the correct definitions.

25. _____ Applications stay at desired temperature longer.

26. _____ Does not penetrate deeply.

27. _____ Temperature must be lower to prevent injury.

28. _____ Heat penetrates more deeply.

29. _____ Higher temperature needed means burns are still a risk.

30. _____ Moist heat applied to small area.

31. _____ Water temperature should be hot (36.6° to 41.1°C [97.8° to 105.9°F]).

32. _____ Tub may be used for applying moist heat to a large area.

a. Dry heat

b. Moist heat

c. Compresses

d. Soaks

TRUE OR FALSE

Circle T for true or F for false. Rewrite all false statements to make them true.

1. **T** **F** The sensor for the pulse oximeter is used only on the fingers.

   _____

   _____

2. **T** **F** The doctor must order oxygen because oxygen is a drug.

   _____

   _____

3. **T** **F** The support worker is responsible for administering oxygen.

   _____

   _____

4. **T** **F** The type of device used to deliver oxygen is decided by the nurse.

   _____

   _____

5. **T** **F** You may remove the cannula or mask used to administer oxygen.

   _____

   _____

6. **T** **F** The oxygen flow is turned off when the person receiving oxygen is out of the room.

   _____

   _____

7. **T** **F** Frequent oral hygiene should be given when the client is receiving oxygen therapy.

   _____

   _____

8. **T** **F** Tracheostomy tubes usually consist of three parts.

   _____

   _____

9. **T** **F** A cover is placed over the tracheostomy tube when outside to prevent dust, insects, and other small particles from entering the stoma.

   _____

   _____

10. **T** **F** Suctioning the upper airway may be done through the mouth and pharynx or the nose and pharynx.

    _____

    _____

11. **T** **F** Suctioning the lower airway may be done through the mouth and pharynx or the nose and pharynx.

    _____

    _____

12. **T** **F** Sterile technique is not required for oro-pharyngeal suctioning.

    _____

    _____

13. **T   F**   You may change the settings on a
                   mechanical ventilator as needed.

     _____

     _____

14. **T   F**   When caring for a client with
                   chest tubes, the drainage system
                   is kept above the level of the
                   client's chest.

     _____

     _____

15. **T   F**   Petrolatum gauze is kept at the
                   bedside to cover the insertion site
                   if a chest tube comes out.

     _____

     _____

FILL-IN-THE-BLANKS

16. What are the three processes that respiratory
     system function involves?

     a. _____

     b. _____

     c. _____

17. Explain how these factors affect oxygen
     needs.

     a. Respiratory system

        _____

     b. Cardiovascular system

        _____

     c. Red blood cell count

        _____

     d. Nervous system

        _____

e. Aging

   _____

f. Exercise

   _____

g. Fever

   _____

h. Pain

   _____

i. Drugs

   _____

j. Smoking

   _____

k. Allergies

   _____

l. Pollutant exposure

   _____

m. Nutrition

   _____

n. Alcohol

   _____

18. Hypoxia is a

    _____ .

    What signs and symptoms would tell you
    the client has hypoxia?

    a. _____

    b. _____

    c. _____

    d. _____

e. _____

f. _____

g. _____

h. _____

i. _____

j. _____

k. _____

l. _____

m. _____

n. _____

o. _____

19. What should you do if the client is wearing dark nail polish when you want to use the pulse oximeter?

_____

20. When a pulse oximeter is used, what should be reported and recorded?

a. _____

b. _____

c. _____

d. _____

e. _____

21. Why are gloves worn when collecting a sputum specimen?

_____

22. Coughing and deep-breathing exercises help

to prevent _____ and

_____ .

23. How is the client instructed to exhale during cough and deep-breathing exercises?

_____

24. Describe each of these oxygen sources.

a. Wall outlet

_____

b. Oxygen tank

_____

c. Oxygen concentrator

_____

25. Describe the following devices used to deliver oxygen.

a. Simple face mask

_____

b. Partial-rebreather mask

_____

c. Nonrebreather mask

_____

d. Venturi mask

_____

26. What should you do if the oxygen humidifier is bubbling?

_____

27. What rules should you follow when handling the tubing for oxygen administration?

    a. _____

    b. _____

    c. _____

28. What fire safety rules should be followed if oxygen is in use?

    a. _____

    b. _____

    c. _____

    d. _____

    e. _____

    f. _____

    g. _____

    h. _____

29. If you observe that the oxygen rate is not set at the rate the nurse stated, what should you do?

    _____

30. Where should the support worker check for signs of irritation from the oxygen cannula or mask?

    _____

31. Why is a humidifier often used in oxygen administration?

    _____

    _____

32. Describe devices used when an artificial airway is needed.

    a. Oro-pharyngeal airway

    _____

    b. Naso-pharyngeal airway

    _____

    c. Endotracheal tube

    _____

    d. Tracheostomy tube

    _____

33. How can you assist the nurse in caring for clients with artificial airways?

    a. _____

    b. _____

    c. _____

    d. _____

34. How can the client with an artificial airway communicate with you?

    _____

    _____

35. What are the parts of a tracheostomy tube?

    a. _____

    b. _____

    c. _____

36. When you are caring for a client with a tracheostomy, you should call the nurse if:

    a. _____ .

    b. _____ .

37. What measures are important to prevent aspiration with a tracheostomy?

    a. _____

    b. _____

    c. _____

    d. _____

    e. _____

    f. _____

    g. _____

38. When assisting with suctioning, the support worker may check the client's pulse, respirations, and pulse oximeter

    _____ ,

    _____ , and

    _____ the procedure.

39. When the support worker is assisting with suctioning, the following should be reported to the nurse:

    a. _____

    b. _____

    c. _____

    d. _____

    e. _____

40. An Ambu bag is used to _____

    _____ before

    _____ to prevent or treat hypoxia.

41. Why is it important to keep the call bell within reach and answer it promptly when you are caring for a client with mechanical ventilation?

    _____

    _____

42. When caring for a client with chest tubes, what information should be observed and reported to the nurse?

    a. _____

    b. _____

    c. _____

    d. _____

    e. _____

    f. _____

43. If you are caring for a client with chest tubes, what should you do if a chest tube comes out, after you call for help?

    a. _____

    b. _____

MULTIPLE CHOICE

Circle the correct answer.

44. A pulse oximeter is used to measure:
    a. oxygen concentration in arterial blood.
    b. the pulse rate.
    c. oxygen concentration in the lungs.
    d. the amount of oxygen in the blood.

45. Which of these procedures may be done by a support worker?
    a. Administering oxygen therapy
    b. Suctioning
    c. Collecting a sputum specimen
    d. Performing tracheostomy care

46. When is the best time to collect a sputum specimen?
    a. At mealtime
    b. Early in the morning
    c. At bedtime
    d. After using mouthwash

47. What position is often preferred by clients with difficulty breathing?
    a. Laying on one side
    b. Supine position
    c. Orthopneic position
    d. Prone position

48. Which of these statements is true about administering oxygen with a face mask?
    a. It irritates the nose and throat.
    b. It makes talking difficult.
    c. The client may eat and drink while it is in place.
    d. Smoking is allowed in the room where the client is sitting.

49. If the support worker is allowed to set up the oxygen administration system, which of the following would not be allowed?
    a. Collect oxygen administration device with the connecting tube.
    b. Attach flowmeter to wall outlet.
    c. Attach humidifier to bottom of flowmeter.
    d. Apply oxygen administration device on the person.

50. When the nurse is giving tracheostomy care, the support worker may be asked to assist when the ties are removed by:
    a. holding the inner cannula in place.
    b. cleaning the outer cannula.
    c. cleaning the stoma.
    d. suctioning the tracheostomy.

51. Which of the following would be the responsibility of the support worker with a client on a mechanical ventilator?
    a. Reset the alarm if it rings.
    b. Use established hand or eye signals for "yes" and "no."
    c. Listen carefully when the person tells what he or she needs.
    d. Both b and c are correct.

52. Mrs. Doronsulic's respiration rate is 34 breaths per minute. This is called:
    a. eupnea.
    b. bradypnea.
    c. tachypnea.
    d. apnea.

53. Which physical condition may most likely contribute to Mrs. Tleen's difficulty breathing?
    a. Diabetes
    b. Epilepsy
    c. Iron-deficiency anemia
    d. Glaucoma

54. Narcotic pain medication can affect breathing by causing:
    a. respiration rates to increase.
    b. thickened mucus in the lungs.
    c. nasal congestion and sinus problems.
    d. suppressed respiration rate and shallower breathing.

MATCHING

Match the tests with the correct descriptions.

55. _____ Measures amount of air moving in and out of lungs

56. _____ Allows doctor to inspect trachea and bronchi

57. _____ Punctures and aspirates air or fluid from the pleura

58. _____ Evaluates changes in lungs

59. _____ Radioactive gas inhaled allows physician to see what areas are not getting air or blood

60. _____ Laboratory test measures amount of oxygen in the blood

a. Chest X-ray

b. Lung scan

c. Bronchoscopy

d. Thoracentesis

e. Pulmonary function tests

f. Arterial blood gases

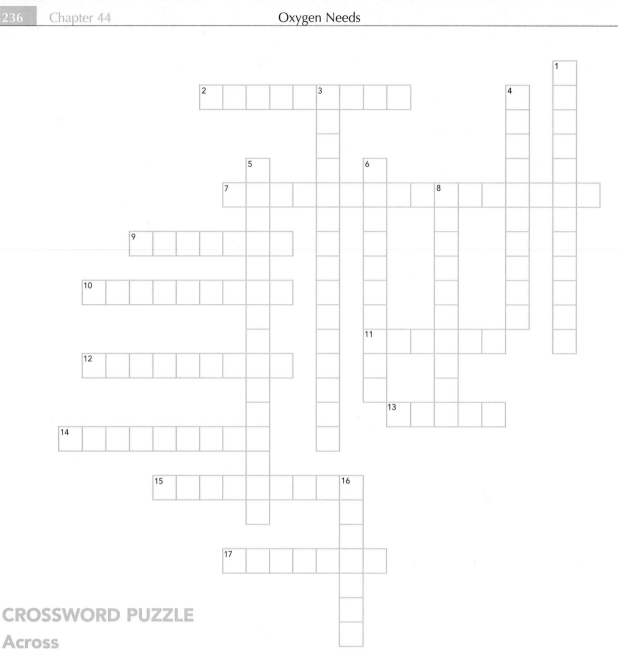

CROSSWORD PUZZLE

Across

2. Rapid breathing; respirations are usually more than 24 per minute
7. Respirations that are rapid and deeper than normal
9. Process of withdrawing or sucking up fluids (secretions)
10. Slow breathing; respirations are fewer than 10 per minute
11. Expectorated mucus
12. Reduced amount of oxygen in the blood
13. Lack or absence of breathing
14. Harmful chemical or substance in the air or water
15. Being able to breathe deeply and comfortably only while sitting or standing
17. Difficult, laboured, or painful breathing

Down

1. Collection of air in the pleural space
3. Escape and collection of fluid in the pleural space (two words)
4. Collection of blood in the pleural space
5. Respirations that are slow, shallow, and sometimes irregular
6. Bloody sputum
8. Process of inserting an artificial airway
16. Sensitivity to a substance that causes the body to react with signs and symptoms

Assisting With the Physical Examination

TRUE OR FALSE

Circle T for true or F for false. Rewrite all false statements to make them true.

1. **T   F**   A nasal spectrum is used to examine the inside of the nose.

   _____

   _____

2. **T   F**   The lithotomy position is used to examine a client's breasts.

   _____

   _____

3. **T   F**   You should always weigh your client before an examination.

   _____

   _____

4. **T   F**   Sims' position is sometimes used to examine the rectum or vagina.

   _____

   _____

5. **T   F**   The examiner (either the doctor or the nurse) will take all of the specimens to the laboratory.

   _____

   _____

FILL-IN-THE-BLANKS

6. What should you explain to the client about the positions used in the examination?

   a. _____

   b. _____

   c. _____

   d. _____

7. Why is the client asked to urinate before an examination?

   a. _____

   b. _____

8. Why is it important to cover a client with a drape during an examination?

   _____

9. Why should a female support worker stay in the examination room with a female client being examined by a male doctor?

   a. _____

   b. _____

10. When a child is being examined, what are two reasons parents may remain in the room?

   a. _____

   b. _____

11. What needs to be done to the examination area after an examination is completed?

   a. Discard _____ .

   b. Replace _____ .

   c. Clean _____ .

   d. Label and send _____ .

MULTIPLE CHOICE

Circle the correct answer.

12. A tuning fork is used to:
   a. examine the mouth.
   b. examine the inside of the nose.
   c. examine the internal structures of the eye.
   d. test hearing.

13. The position the client is usually in for an examination of the abdomen is the:
   a. lithotomy position.
   b. knee-chest position.
   c. Sims' position.
   d. supine position.

14. The client needs to void before an examination to ensure that:
   a. the examiner can feel the abdominal cavity.
   b. a full bladder does not change the normal position and shape of the organs.
   c. none of the above
   d. a and b

15. The knee-chest position is used to examine the:
   a. rectum.
   b. abdomen.
   c. breasts.
   d. chest.

16. You can provide your client with privacy during an examination by:
   a. ensuring that your client is undressed for the examination.
   b. closing the door to his or her room.
   c. letting the doctor or nurse explain the examination.
   d. asking everyone to leave the room even if the client has asked for a family member to be present.

MATCHING

Match each description with the correct position.

17. _____ Hips down to edge of table, knees flexed, feet in stirrups

18. _____ Lying on side with upper leg flexed

19. _____ Lying on back with legs together or knees flexed

20. _____ Kneeling with body supported on knees and chest

a. Supine

b. Lithotomy

c. Knee-chest

d. Sims'